Resistance Band Training

How to Handle Resistance Bands for Your Workout

Table of Contents

Medical Disclaimer:

You should consult your physician before starting any exercise routine.

If you have any questions about any medical matter you should consult a doctor.

If during your workout you suffer from any medical condition you should seek immediate medical attention.

The recommendations in this document are for educational purpose only. The exercises contained in this book are for healthy individuals 18 years or older.

Before starting your exercise routine you should make sure that your resistance bands are in perfect condition. Always warm-up before you start exercising. It is recommended to use yoga mat to perform exercises with resistance loop bands.

If you experience dizziness or shortness of breath you should stop exercising and consult your physician.

Introduction

Resistance bands are amongst the most unique items that you can utilize when it comes to working out. Great resistance bands can help you add a little bit of extra pressure to a workout, thus requiring a bit of extra effort to complete different movements. These bands are easy to handle and won't require you to get anything far too costly or otherwise too heavy to handle.

Today you can use resistance bands for all sorts of workouts. This guide will help you see how to make a resistance band workout run for you.

You will learn about the different movements and exercises that you can do in your workout. You will also learn about what you can do to make a resistance band workout more efficient based on how to get a workout to run with the right support surfaces while also ensuring that your bands are strong enough to handle your great workouts.

The exercises that are covered in this guide include several that will help you out with different movements all around the body. You can use this guide to learn about arm and leg movements and even a few that will help you with your abs. Each of these exercises is fully described in detail to help you understand how to make this work for you.

Working with resistance bands can prove to be one of the best things that you can do when it comes to getting a strong workout. This guide will show you how user-friendly these resistance bands are.

If you don't own resistance bands yet, there are plenty set to choose from available for sale on Amazon. I would like to recommend you a set of bands which includes long bands and short bands with different accessories to spice up your workout. Koyto Sports which is the seller of this products offers 25% discount for this set (and all of their other products) with promo code 3U66RIDG for all readers of my book. Just click the link below to check it out.

https://www.amazon.com/dp/B01DT0F04S

Chapter 1 – What Are Resistance Bands?

It is truly amazing how resistance bands can do more for your workouts. But before you start working on your resistance band workout routine, you have to first understand what makes these bands so special and worthwhile. Resistance bands are among the most unique items that you can use when working out.

Resistance bands are large and flexible and elastic. You will hold on to the band (since it is supported by a part of your body) while working out as you pull it in and out for you to make all your necessary movements.

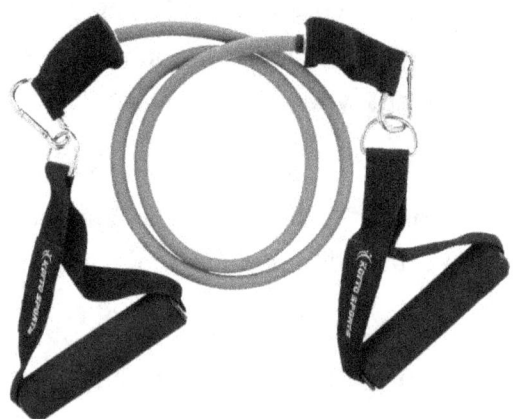

These bands are often made of out latex and rubber among other flexible materials. Depending on what you have, you might find your bands to be in one of many colors. The companies that make these bands will sell their products in different resistance levels that are designated by a series of colors with some representing stronger ones.

In some cases you can find handles on the ends of these bands. These are to help you handle your bands and keep control of your workouts and your movements as you use them.

You can make use of resistance bands in a variety of ways:

- You can add them to a lifting machine.
- You can have the bands supported by your feet.
- You can also hold the bands with your hands and use them to add a bit of extra pressure to some of your movements.
- A band can also be supported by a door or other surface through an anchor. You will have to get this to work with a steady and stable door for it to work.

The resistance band is a material that can make a difference when it comes to working out. In fact, resistance bands can be found in many sizes, weights and pressure levels.

The overall amount of pressure that will be generated by a band will vary based on how tense and even how large it is. It is difficult to figure out the precise amount of weight or pressure that is being added but you will certainly feel it as you are getting your workout completed.

In fact, the pressure that is added is typically measured in ranges on each band, thus meaning that every movement that you have could potentially come with a different level of pressure. For instance, a lighter band can offer from 2 to 5 extra pounds of resistance. A much larger or heavy duty option will work with about 15 to 20 extra pounds. It's obviously tough to get a precise measurement of the added resistance, but each band should at least offer some kind of range that you can work with.

Some resistance bands may also be shorter than others and are designed for exercises that are a little more restrained in terms of how your body will be moved. This is to help you work a little harder to get your muscles to be triggered and move properly.

How Will Your Body Be Impacted

The impacts that you will feel as you are using resistance bands are certainly important to see by working with resistance bands:

- You can improve your overall range of motion.
- Your flexibility can upgrade as you will be using more movements relating to pulling items.
- Your stamina can also be boosted as it will be easier to handle one of these bands than a typical set of free weights.
- You can work with all kinds of body parts as well. You can use resistance bands on your arms and legs and even your abs.

Why Use Resistance Bands?

There are many other good reasons why you should be using resistance bands for a workout:

- It doesn't cost much for you to get one of these resistance bands. Many of these bands can cost around ten to twenty dollars each.

- Resistance bands come in a number of resistance levels. These include ones with light or heavy resistance levels.
- You could use as many of these bands as desired if you want to add a bit of a challenge.
- By using one of these items, you will get a full-body workout going. You can use a band on any part of the body.
- These are safe to use in that you can get one of these handled without being at much of a risk of breaking apart.
- There's no need to get any outside equipment used when getting resistance bands ready. These are flexible and compact enough to where you can use them anywhere without gathering any other weights. Of course, you can always add these weights to a piece of equipment like free weights if you are interested. There's a chapter later in this guide that lists info on how to use it with free weights plus another for treadmill use.

With all of these points in mind, it is important to get the right workouts ready when trying to get the most out of your workout. Much of this book is dedicated to helping you get into some effective exercises with resistance bands but before we get to that, let's look at some pointers for when you're trying to prepare for a good workout with resistance bands.

Chapter 2 – Workout Preparations

As great as resistance bands can be, there are a few things that you need to do before you can get your workout ready. You must make sure you are prepared well enough so it won't be too hard for you to get the most out of your resistance bands. This is regardless of whether you plan on working with shorter or longer bands.

1. Make sure you are dressed properly.

You need to wear proper workout clothes to help improve your overall range of motion. This is especially since resistance band exercises will require you to move your body quite well. The pictures of assorted exercises that you will see in this guide will help you figure out what you wear for your workout.

2. Get a proper anchor.

You need to get an anchor for your resistance bands so you can get it secured to a surface in the case that you are not able to get your feet or hands to work as a natural anchor. A few of the exercises you will go through during a workout actually require you to use a good anchor.

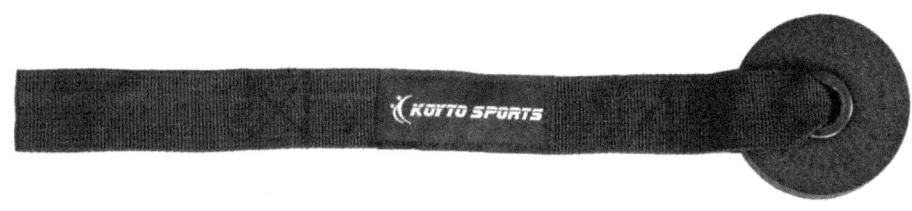

Anchors can be found in a variety of forms. Some of them can be hung up on a door or other surface. They may include traditional hooks but some options made of fabric can be used to create strong grips for you to use.

The anchor is used for when you need additional support for the workout and when you are doing an exercise that doesn't entail your feet being used to keep the band down at the floor. It should not be used as a full substitute for your handles

3. Check the handles on your bands.

The handles on your bands will be important as they will help you to keep a good grip on your bands while working out. Good padded handles are perfect as they ensure that you'll have enough of a grip to work with. Also, a padded handle will be less likely to slip apart while you're working out.

You can also choose to wear gloves for your workout if needed. Good workout gloves can come with padding materials or grooves to help you keep a strong grip on anything you are holding onto.

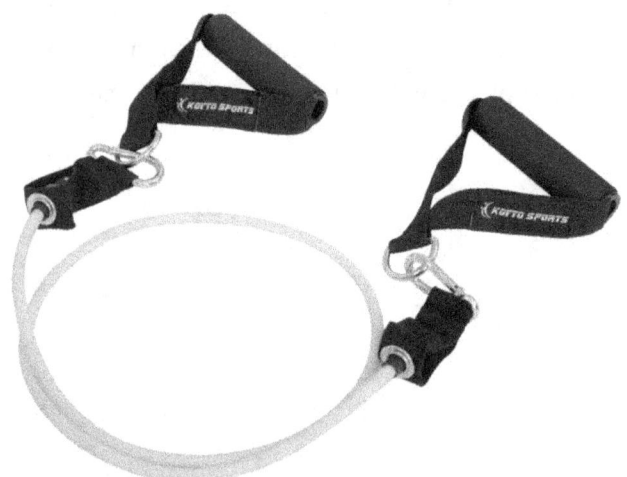

4. Look to see that your bands are secure.

While elastic resistance bands can be amazingly powerful and effective for your workout, there are often times when they might suffer from fatigue. This fatigue can come from the stretching motions that keep coming about. Over time a band might be at risk of tearing apart.

Check your bands to see that they don't have any tears or fatigue marks on them. You might have to get new ones if your current bands are wearing out and are at an increased risk of tearing apart.

5. Watch for the positions of your bands when making them work.

Many of the exercises you'll see here involve the use of an anchor or your feet to keep your band secure. You'll have to keep the spot that is being pushed down or anchored in the middle as well as possible. This is to create an even balance so the bands will be used right.

With all these points in mind, it's time to get into the many workouts you can use when getting resistance bands to work to your advantage. Let's look and see what you can do with your bands.

Chapter 3 – Arm Workouts

You can strengthen various muscles with your arms through the exercises listed in this chapter.

These workouts are done best with about three sets on each one. You can use ten or so reps on each set although some of the exercises might require fewer reps due to how extensive they might be.

Curls

Curls are important arm exercises in that you will be moving your arms up and down while lifting something. The arms will be all the way down at the start.

For these curls, you will have to get a resistance band supported by your feet. You can then hold onto the ends of the band with both your hands.

The particular curls that you can use are divided into three different forms:

Standing Bicep Curls

This basic bicep exercise works to improve these important arm muscles.

Standing Bicep Curls

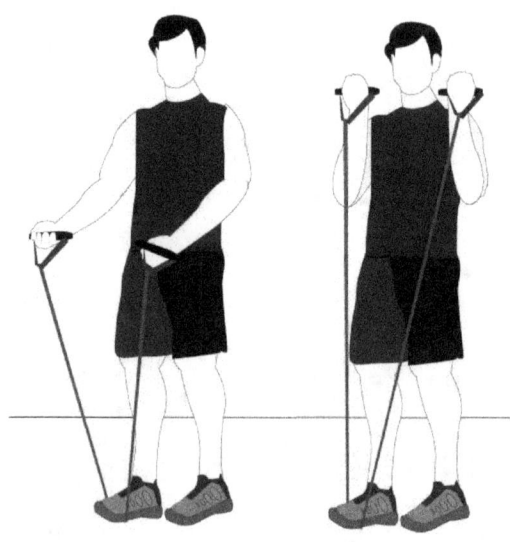

1. Keep your arms to your sides at the start while your palms face towards your body as you are holding onto the band.

2. Holding the band with both hands, move the lower arms upward while keeping your upper arms and elbows still.

3. The wrist will naturally rotate as you do this. The wrist should be facing your shoulder as you move all the way up.

4. Keep your shoulders are tight as possible when lifting.

Work with about 10 to 20 reps in each session. You can use one or both arms at the same time but it's best to use the same number of reps for each arm.

Hammer Curls

This requires a little more concentration. You must make sure your elbows are in a stationary position at all times:

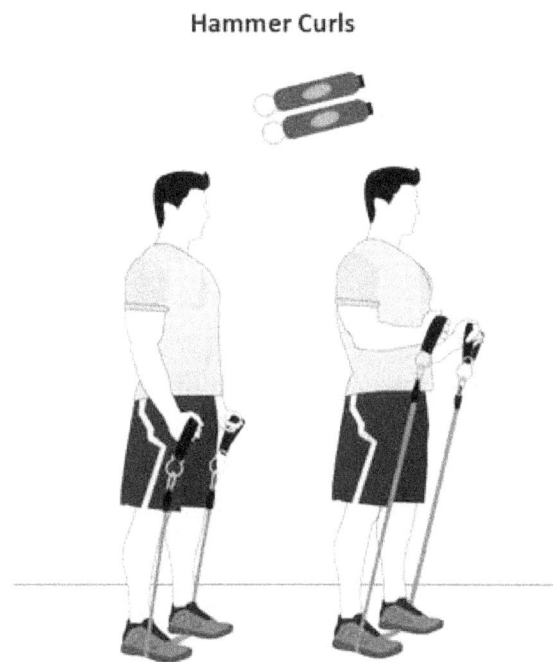

Hammer Curls

1. Grab your bands with them around your ankles. As you do this, grip the handles. Allow the fingers to be inside the strap with the thumbs on the outside parts of the handles.

2. Keep your feet at a hip's width apart from each other.

3. Pull the handles up and bend the arms to where they are at your chest's height.

Overhead Bicep Curls

This requires the use of an anchor to hang the band over your head.

Overhead Bicep Curls

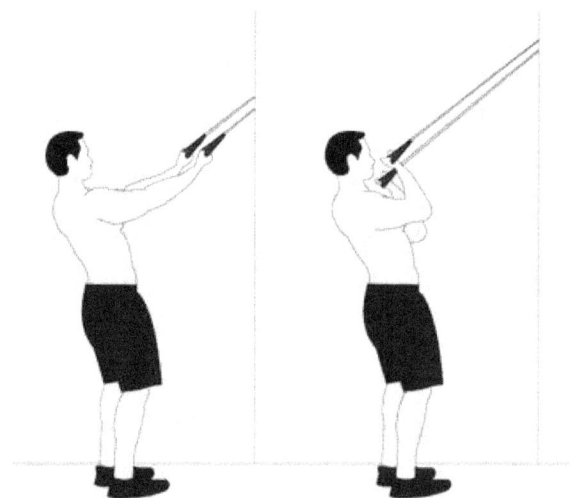

1. Secure your resistance band onto an anchor. It helps to use a door anchor that can be placed on top of a door that you have closed shut.

2. Step away from the door to a point where you can feel tension in your band.

3. Hold onto the band with your palm facing your body. The arm should be fully stretched outward.

4. Complete the curls by bringing your handle towards your shoulder without moving your upper arm.

Deltoid Flies

The deltoid fly is designed to help you build upon your shoulder muscles. This works well with a shorter band that you don't have to step on.

Deltoid Flies

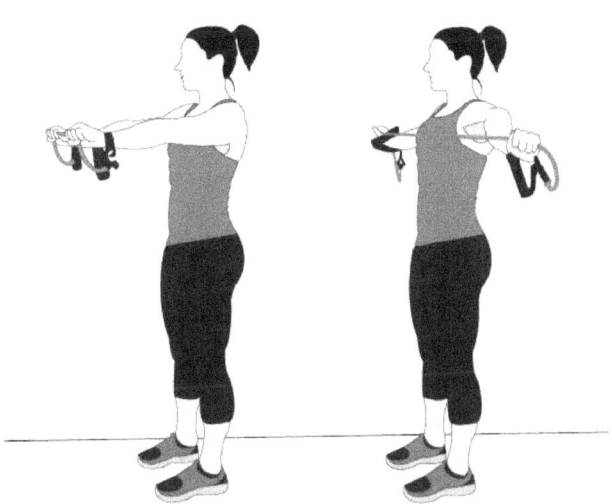

1. Keep your feet shoulder-width apart.

2. Hold onto the band with the arms on the sides.

3. Raise the arms up in a perpendicular fashion. They must be aligned with the body.

4. Hold the arms out to where your body creates a perfect T-like shape.

5. Return the arms down to the sides

This should work for 15 to 20 reps at a time. You can add free weights if desired.

Shoulder Presses

This also works well for the shoulders.

1. Stand on the band like with the deltoid flies exercise.

2. Keep your palms up as you hold onto the band. Get the palms to move up to the pectorals.

3. Move the hands up straight to where you are creating a loose I-shape. The elbows can bend out by a small bit as you are doing so.

4. Move the hands back to the chest and repeat.

This can work for 10 to 15 reps. Also, make sure the back is straight and the palms are up so you can get a full range of motion on this exercise.

Shoulder Presses

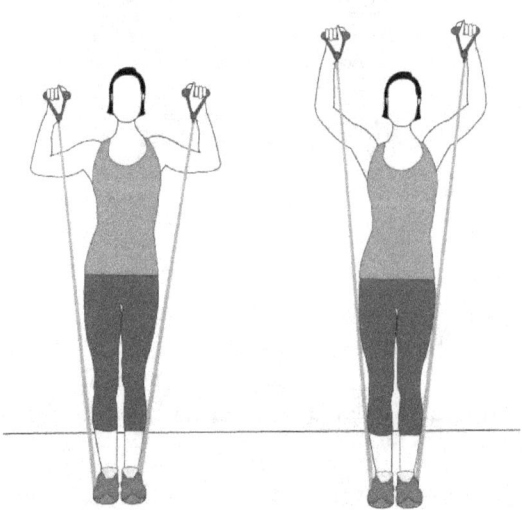

Tricep Extensions

You can use this workout option to stretch your triceps. This requires the band being placed on your back.

Tricep Extensions

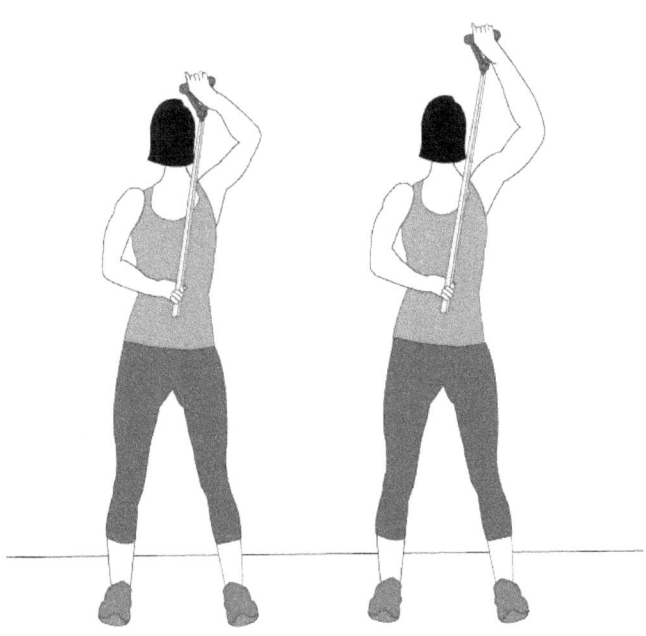

1. Support the middle of the band with your feet and stretch the band over your back to create an X-shape.

2. Hold onto the handles near your neck with your palms facing your body. Your elbows should be outward as high up as the top of your head.

3. Stretch your arms up all the way, forming straight lines with each arm. Make sure the arms are parallel to each other and that the elbows are locked.

4. Move back to the initial position.

This can work for ten to twelve repetitions in a set.

Overhead Tricep Extensions

You can also use an overhead form of the tricep extension with an anchor used at the top of a door or other surface.

1. Keep one foot ahead of the other at the start and hold onto the band with the palms facing each other. They should be near the top of the head.

2. Keeping your legs and feet still, move your arms outward in a parallel fashion while holding the band. The arms should be out straight and the palms should still face each other.

3. Move the arms back into the original position.

Tricep Extensions

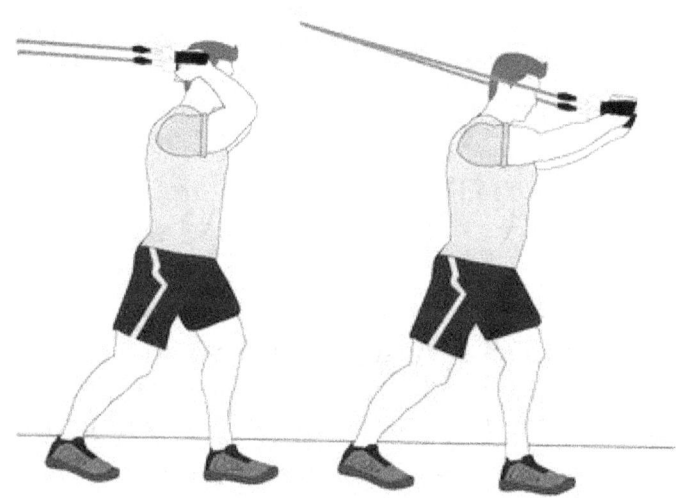

Anti-Rotation Press

This is a workout that focuses on the shoulders.

Anti-Rotation Press

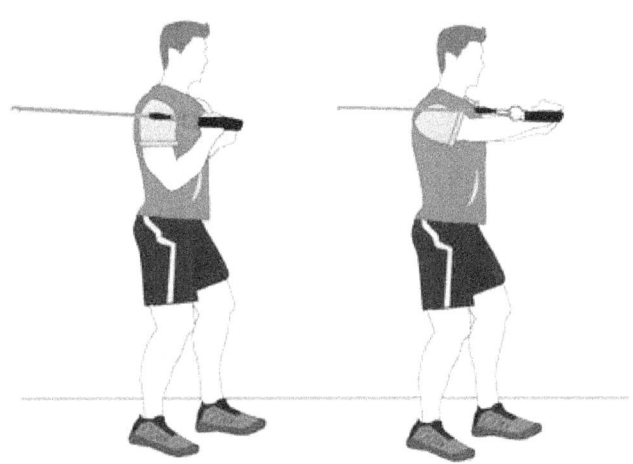

1. Secure the band on a door or anchor aligned with your chest.

2. Hold the band with your hands clasped together next to your chest.

3. Step slightly from the door until you start to feel a bit of tension from the band.

4. Bend the knees by a bit and then extend your arms forward, holding for about ten seconds.

5. After this, return your arms back to your chest.

This can work for three reps in a set. You should do three sets for the best results.

Chest Press

You can use this to target your biceps. This also requires an anchor for you to use to make it work right.

1. Anchor the band on a door or wall surface at the chest level. You will have to stand with your back facing the door while holding the band with each hand. Keep the elbows bent so the fists are in front of your chest.

2. Step forward while holding the bands. Move forward until you start to feel a bit of tension in your band.

3. Keep one leg back and move forward by a small bit with your hips doing the moving. Keep the feet as flat on the ground as possible.

4. Push your hands forward and then bring your elbows back to the starting position.

    This works best when you get twelve to fifteen reps in each set.

Chest Press

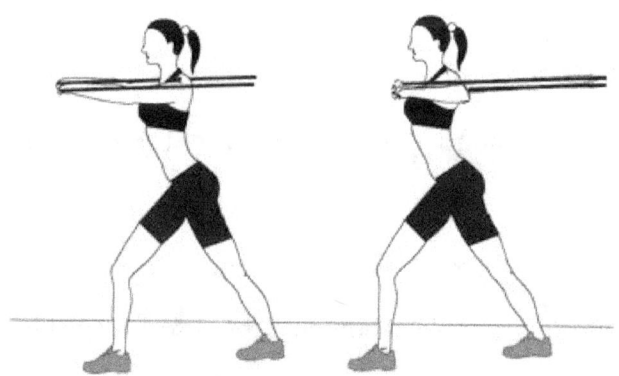

Chapter 4 – Leg Exercises

This chapter is about the leg exercises that you can use when getting a workout with resistance bands to be to your advantage. You can do these as a means of not only improving your leg muscles but also with enhancing your overall sense of balance.

Most of these exercises are designed to help with the upper legs although all parts of the legs can benefit from resistant band workouts.

Squats

Squats are exercises that require you to bend your legs and knees down and then back up. This is a basic type of exercise but it can be useful if managed properly.

Squats

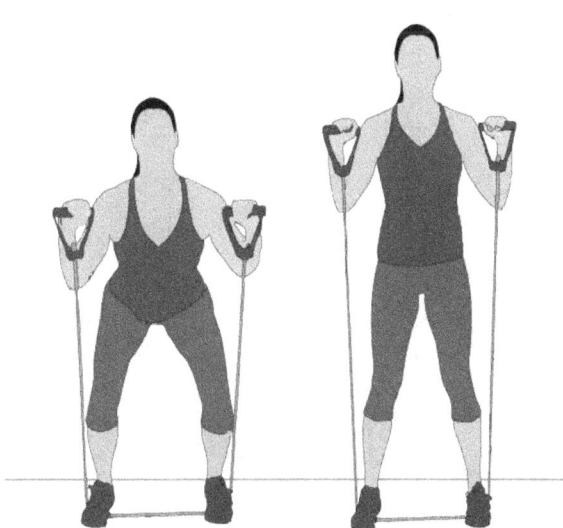

1. Keep the toes a bit towards the outside of the body. Allow the feet to point away from each other.

2. Hold the resistance band behind your back, keeping the ends up above or at your shoulders. Make sure the handles are at the same part all throughout the exercise.

3. Keeping your back straight, bend your knees down evenly. Make sure the butt sticks out while you are doing this. Do not move your hands too much when bending down.

4. Push back up to the starting position. Push down on the heels and make sure they do not move up.

5. This can work for about ten reps on each set. Try and do three sets if possible.

The muscles you'll be working on will vary based on how far apart the feet are. If your wide are wide apart then you will be working more on your hamstrings. If they are closer to each other then you will be working on your quads.

Lunges

Lunges work in that you will bend your legs as you move in a forward position and then go back to the starting point. This can be done with one leg being used at a time.

Lunges Excersise

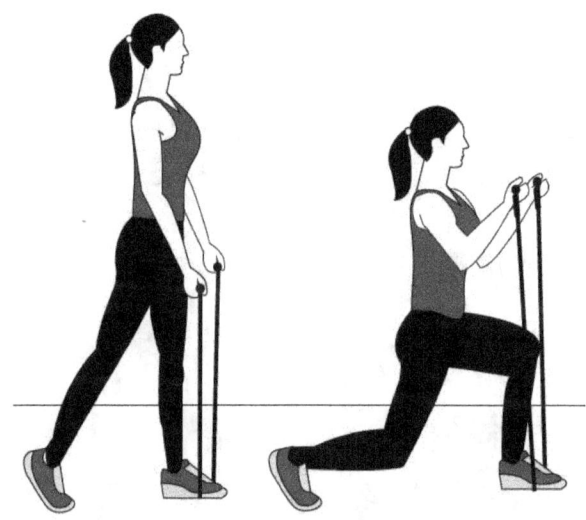

1. Start by stepping on the band with one foot while the ends are held right around your shoulders.

2. Keep the opposite leg behind the one that is stepping on the band.

3. Bend the leg standing on the band to where the knee sticks outward. Try and get a right angle formed.

4. The other leg should bend down to where the knee and the lower part is flat on the floor. Again, this needs to have a right angle.

5. Push up with your back straight and firm and move back into the original position.

Make sure you keep your back and head in the same position during each rep. You must also make sure you use the same number of reps and sets for each leg.

Kickbacks

The kickback works more on the glutes. This exercise requires you to be on the ground to help you with getting your movements handled properly.

1. Put your hands and knees on the floor while keeping the band on the bottom of one of your feet. The handles can be hooked to a surface in front of you.

2. Extend the leg that has the band on it back. Move it in a straight line and try to squeeze the glute at this point.

3. Move the leg back to the starting position.

Again, this is a workout that is best when you do the same number of reps for each leg.

kickback Excersise

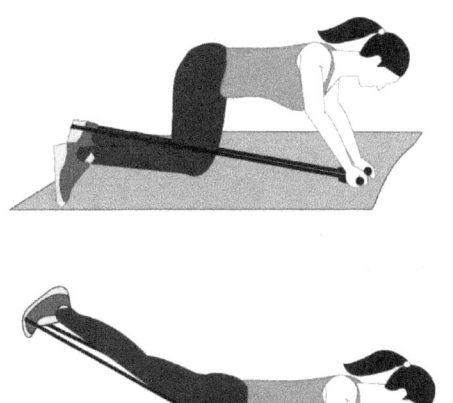

Calf Raises

This is an exercise designed for use on the lower legs. Specifically, this one works for the calves.

1. Secure your band with a low hook near your feet. This works well if you use a door hook.

2. Grab your handles and keep them near the hips with your hands facing the hips.

3. Extend your calves as you gently lift the heels up.

4. The band's pressure should be felt as you are lifting your calves off of the ground.

5. Move back in a gentle motion.

Make sure your legs and back are perfectly straight so you will get the full range of motion on this exercise.

Calf Raises

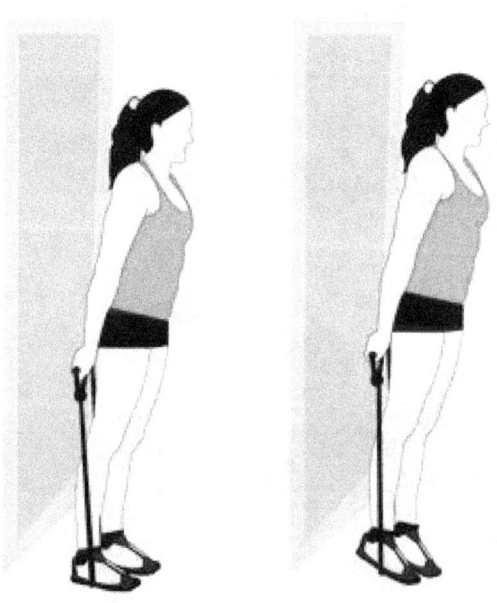

Lying Hamstring Curls

Lying hamstring curls require you to get on a soft surface and to move your legs up as you bend at the knees. This exercise will work well on your hamstrings.

Lying Hamstring Curls

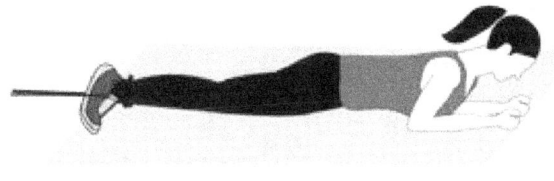

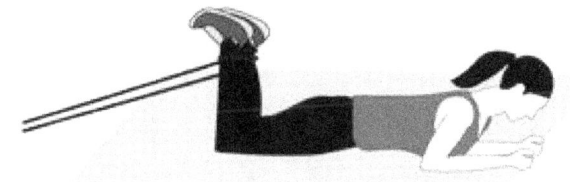

1. Secure your resistance band to a door anchor while using a series of straps on your ankles.

2. Position your body to the ground on a pad while keeping your back flat.

3. Bend your legs together while moving the heels around the buttocks.

4. Relax the calves so they will not make the exercise any harder to complete. This is also to help you keep a straight line going while lifting.

5. Keep your hips down while lifting.

6. Move your legs back down after completing a lift.

This can work for about ten to fifteen reps in a set. Make sure each one results in you creating a right angle while lifting.

Although that last leg exercise can work for both legs at once, most of these workouts for your legs will target just one leg at a time. This is different form the arm workouts that work with both arms. Be sure to plan your workouts appropriately so it will be easier for you to get a workout to run properly and to evenly target all parts of your body.

It is true that there aren't as many leg-oriented exercises for you to work with but these will certainly work well when do properly. One other idea for your legs involves using these on a treadmill; this will be discussed in a few chapters from now.

Chapter 5 – Ab Workouts

The abdominal muscles are among the most targeted muscles in the human body when it comes to workouts. It's all about making it easier for the body to handle a better physical look and to also keep all that annoying and stubborn belly fat from getting in the way of that good look you've always wanted.

Resistance bands can be used to target your abdominal muscles. Here are a few of the best steps you can use when getting ab workouts to run for you.

A quite note: Keep the bands that you're using as even as possible so you can get a good workout. Also, you need to keep your back straight to get the best range of motion out of these exercises.

Rowboat

The rowboat exercise requires you to sit down while working out. This is used to create a rowing motion similar to what you'd have on a traditional boat or even with a rowing machine.

Rowboat

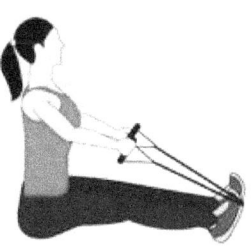

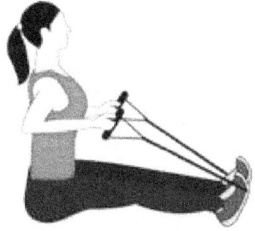

1. Sit down with the knees bent forward by a small bit. Keep the heels on the floor and put the feet at least a foot apart from one another.

2. Get the bands looped around the arches of your feet.

3. Bend the elbows about 90 degrees as you hold onto the handles.

4. Lean the torso back by 45 degrees and move the handles back to the shoulders. Try and hold this position for a few seconds if you can.

5. Move slightly forward at the hips as the arms are extended.

6. Extend the arms behind your body. Again, the elbows have to be close to the body.

You should do about ten to fifteen reps to make this work.

Crouching Tiger

This requires you to keep your hands and feet at the ground with the rest of your body moving upward.

Crouching Tiger

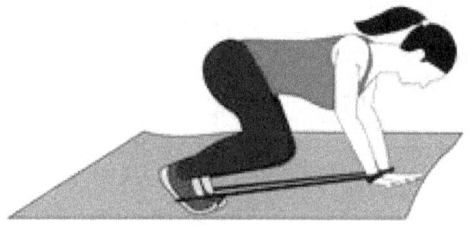

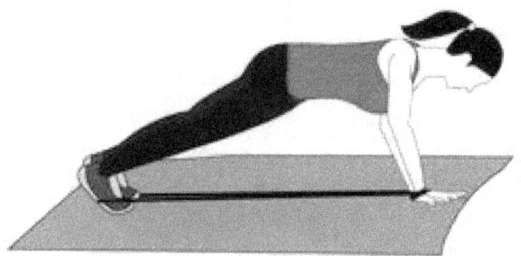

1. Stand with your feet apart at the hips' distance.

2. Keep the middle of your feet on the band. Cross the band in front of you once.

3. Crouch downward and get into a push-up position. The hands should be flat on the floor at this point.

4. Extend the arms outward with the palms under the shoulders.

5. Bend the knees down with your rear sticking outward. Get your body to move closer to the ground at this point. The knees should be right over the floor but not touching.

6. Straighten the legs and move back up to the original push-up position.

This one can work for about ten reps. Again, keep your back straight as well as possible during the entire workout.

Chapter 6 – Working With Weights and Exercise Balls

You don't have to use any extra weights or other pieces of equipment with your resistance bands but they could still help you out if you are careful with them. You can add resistance bands to weights if you want to add an extra bit of resistance.

This is great if you are focused on a strength training program. A resistance band can add an extra amount of pressure onto the weights to help you get them lifted properly.

The ways how you can get these weights adjusted with resistance bands can be rather varied and important for your use. You can add the handles to your hands as you are working with different weights that you will lift with your hands, for instance. You can also add them to a leg workout machine to create an extra layer of resistance on a squatting machine or other item that targets your leg muscles.

Working With Weights

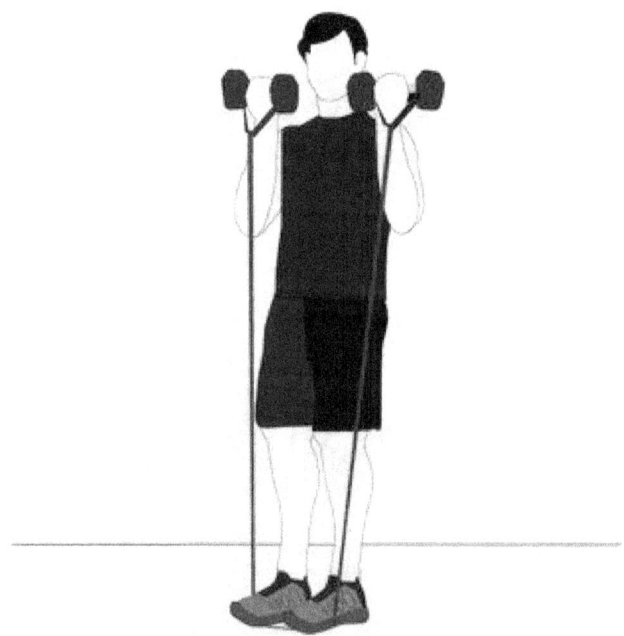

As this picture shows, it is easy to use these resistance bands with free weights. You will have to stand on the band in order to make them work though.

There are a few pointers that must be used if you want to add resistance bands to any weights that you're lifting:

- Look to see that you have a firm grip on the bands. Keep the handles in your hands or any other secure items for as long as possible.

- Make sure there's a strong foundation to keep the bands in place. You might have to stand on the bands or you might need to get an anchor to work for them while lifting.

- Only lift whatever you are actually capable of lifting. You need to build muscle mass before you can actually get a good series of items lifted carefully enough.

Meanwhile, you can always use an exercise ball with your resistance bands. This can work with your body being supported by an exercise ball while using resistance bands or you can add the ball on top of a resistance band.

This is used to help you primarily strengthen your core muscles while working out. In addition to lifting with your resistance bands, you are also trying to strengthen your core by keeping the ball stable and in the same position at all times.

Exercise Balls

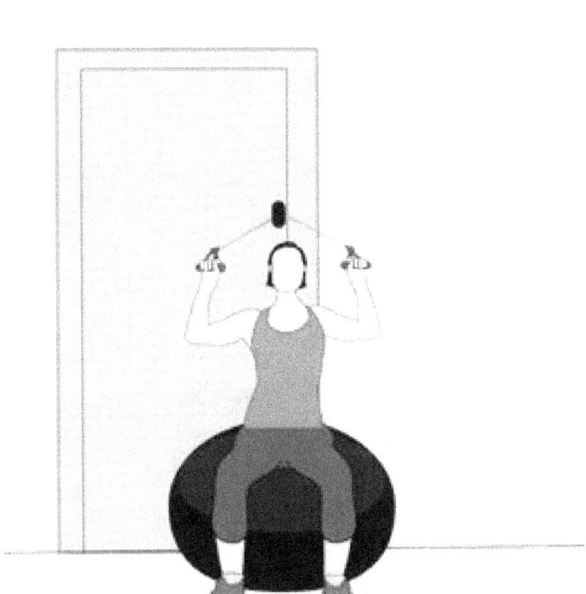

This can be a great option for a workout that adds a bit of a challenge but at the same time you have to be careful when doing exercises on an exercise ball. The ball must be properly inflated and situated on a surface where it will not slip. This should give you the opportunity to keep your muscles triggered the right way.

It is also best to use resistance bands that have handles on them. This is to give you a little bit of extra support for getting the bands to work for you.

There might be times when you could get your resistance bands secured onto the sides of an exercise ball. However, you'd have to buy a separate exercise ball that has small handles or loops on the sides to ensure that you'll have something that is easy to lift with while keeping this as controlled as possible.

Working with weights can always add a good deal of pressure for when you're lifting something. Be sure to look carefully when getting your bands ready so you'll find something that is stronger and efficient.

Chapter 7 – Exercises With Short Resistance Bands

You might think that resistance bands are always going to be a little longer in length than most other pieces of equipment but you can also use a shorter set of bands. Shorter bands are often used with wrist or ankle straps to make them easier to handle so they will stay close to your body during a workout.

You can use these shorter bands to perfect a variety of different exercises. These exercises are perfect for when you are looking to get a carefully controlled workout.

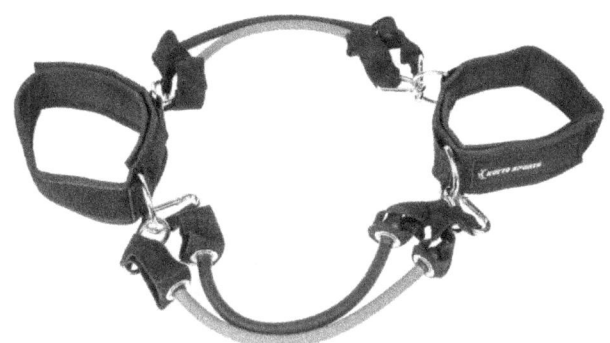

Side Stepping

Side stepping is a great exercise for strengthening your hips.

1. Put ankle straps (with short tubes attached) around your ankles. You can choose from one of various resistance levels for your bands including 10 to 15 pounds to add a challenge.

2. Bend your knees by a small bit while the feet are hip-width apart.

3. Slide one foot over to the side and then slide the pivot foot over towards that other foot to create the same stance you originally had.

4. Repeat about 10 to 20 times in one direction.

5. Repeat in the opposite direction with the same number of reps.

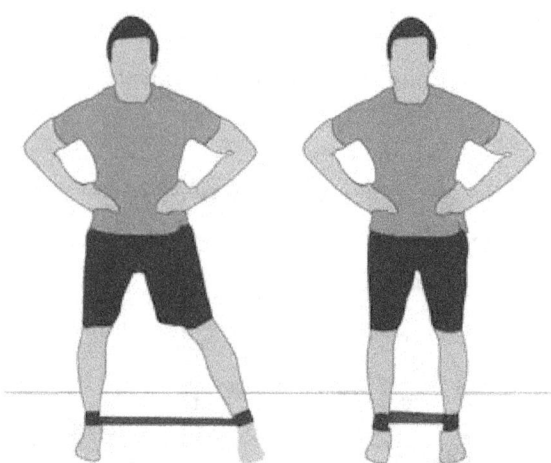

Monster Walk

This is loosely related to side stepping in that this workout for short resistance bands allows you to exercise your hip muscles and upper legs.

1. Look a short band around the knees.

2. Bend your knees down with the rear outward to allow it to keep your balance as you are walking. Keep your feet apart by the hips like in the side stepping exercise. Keep your arms down on the sides of your body too.

3. Step forward at 45 degrees with one leg. Keep your knees bent at the same position while doing so.

4. Move your other leg forward at 45 degrees in the opposite direction.

5. Keep moving your legs outward in the same position for about 10 to 20 feet.

This can work with either leg being used as the dominant leg but you should try to keep it steady and consistent.

Monster Walk

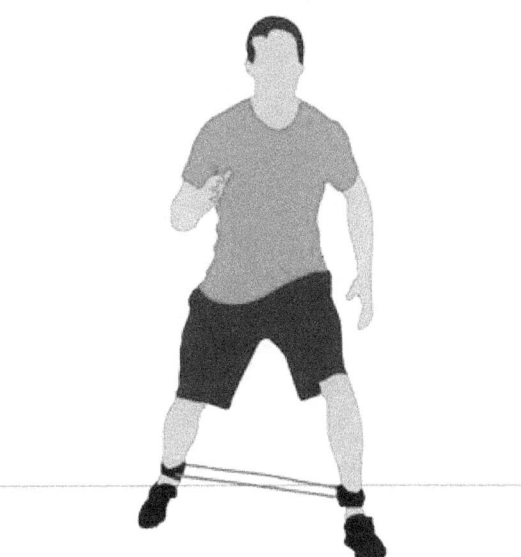

Standing Abductor

This is used to target the inner thighs. If used carefully, it will be easier for your body to target the muscles and get a better range of motion.

1. Secure the band onto an anchor. Use a door anchor for the best results as it can create a good surface that will support the band.

2. Keep the other end attached to ankle strap on your leg.

3. Stand in a wide stance with the ankle that the band is attached to further from the anchor than the other ankle.

4. Slide the ankle past your other one as you move it closer to the anchor. After this, move the ankle back outward from the rest of your body.

5. Move back to the starting position.

Do this for 12 to 15 reps on each leg. This works best if you can squeeze your thighs as you do this. This is to trigger an added amount of movement in those muscles and to help you use them properly while lifting. This should be a suitable exercise for a short band as it will improve how well you can keep your thighs working in tight distances.

Standing Abductor

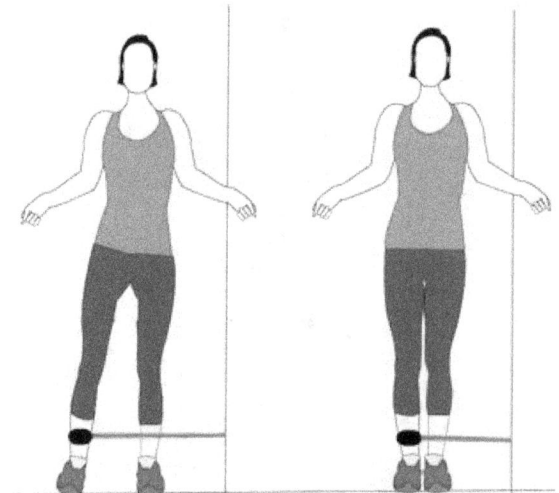

Pull Downs

A pull down can be used to help you with stretching your arms and helping to support your elbows to be stronger.

1. Hold onto the band with your arms straight and the cuffs on your hands.

2. Hold the band overhead and then pull it out until it gets to the front of your chest.

3. Hold the short band in front of the chest for a second and then bring it back to an overhead position.

4. Try and squeeze your outside back muscles while performing this move.

You can do about fifteen of these moves at a time.

Pull Downs

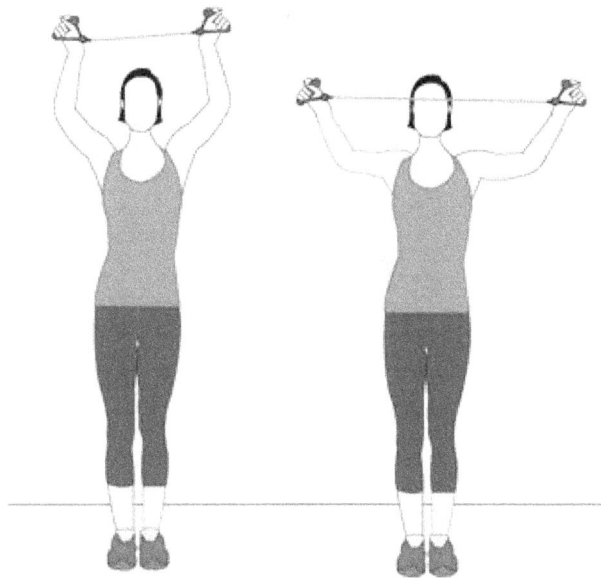

Side Bends

Another exercise that involves handling a short band with your hands, this is used to help you lengthen your waist muscles. This in turn may help you out when trying to get belly fat under control.

1. Keep your feet apart by the hips.

2. Hold your band overhead.

3. Stretch your hip out towards your side as you start to feel a stretching sensation in your stomach muscles.

4. Keep your navel aligned along the spine as well as possible.

5. Move your body back to the original position.

Do this for about twenty reps on each side of the body. Try and keep the arms out in a Y-shape when you are straight so the workout will be efficient enough for you to handle.

By using shorter bands, you can get a more concentrated workout running by using bands that can be easily handled by your ankles or wrists and hands. When used properly, you can get this to work well.

Side Bends

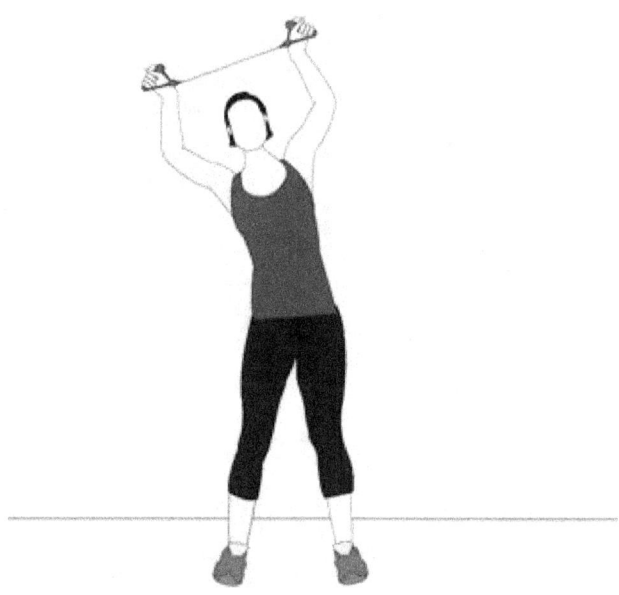

Chapter 7 – Key Tips

As great as the exercises used in a resistance band workout can be, there are a few important tips that you need to use in order to make your workout effective. You must be certain when using resistance bands that you are careful with making it work.

Look For Stable Surfaces

You have to make sure that the surfaces that will support your resistance bands are sturdy and strong. For instance, you need to keep your feet steady and secure if you're going to have it supported by your feet.

There are times when you can use an anchor attached to a door or rod or other hard surface. As you read earlier, an anchor can be perfect for use but you must make sure that anything you use your anchor on is stable enough to where the anchor won't be at risk of tearing off. Only keep an anchor on a steady surface like a strong door or walled surface among other things. Don't place it on something that could tear apart.

This is especially important if you plan on using an exercise ball. An exercise ball should be grooved and textured well enough to where it will stay on the floor without being at risk or slipping around. Of course, the ball should be flexible enough to where it could move slightly if you don't keep it steady. Be sure when making this work that you look for something strong to handle for your resistance ball needs.

Use Your Bands Carefully

As strong and flexible as resistance bands can be, you must be careful when getting these ready for your use. The problem with some bands is that they might wear out over time, what with all that pressure that you can apply onto your bands.

With this in mind, you need to be cautious. You have to make sure you stretch your bands properly and in accordance with your workout routine so you will not put too much undue stress onto them.

As mentioned earlier in this guide, you need to check on your bands before working out to ensure that your bands won't wear out. While working out, take note of any unusual sounds that might come from your band. Any odd stretching sounds or cracking noises might be signs of a band potentially wearing out.

Keep your bands dry if possible too. Sweat is common during any workout but you must dry off your bands so they won't bear with any sweat that can potentially wear out their bodies and keep them from being so flexible and powerful.

Check Your Surroundings

Resistance bands require you to put in a full range of motion no matter what kind of exercise you perform. With that in mind, you need to use these resistance bands in a responsible manner to where you can easily use them to move your muscles without obstructions.

Avoid using resistance bands in spots where there are far too many things in the way. You need to keep your space for working out clear and open so it won't be hard for you to get that workout running right.

Avoid Slippery Skin

Your skin needs to be fully dry before using any of these resistance bands. This is to prevent them from slipping off and possibly harming someone during a workout.

You should wipe off any lotions you've used or any sweat that might have come about during a workout. This should be done to help you stay comfortable and keep the risks that come with a workout under control.

Make sure you have a good workout towel to help you dry off as well. A towel can be used on your resistance bands too.

Review Each Band

The amazing thing about today's resistance bands is that they are made in many forms with different colors, handle features, lengths, resistance levels and much more. There's a particular type of band that is available for just about everyone out there.

Still, you need to be cautious when getting a good band ready. You have to review each band that you are interested in using so you will have something that you know won't be too hard to use.

You have to review each band by looking to see that whatever you have is easy to hold and won't be at risk of snapping or wearing out among other threats. You have to also see that a band has a resistance level that you are comfortable with.

Check the handles if there are any. If there are no handles then you should look to see that the band has a smooth and comfortable texture that you can easily handle. Choose something that isn't going to put too much stress on you so it will be easier for you to make it work.

Your resistance bands can be the key to a great workout. You have to make sure whatever you are working with is managed properly to make it easier for you to get the most out of any workout you have while still being very easy to use for your workout demands.

Conclusion

The great part of working with resistance bands is that it's amazingly easy to complete a good workout with these items. By using resistance bands, you can target every part of your body. This can help you with getting your body to be conditioned quite well.

The effects you'll get out of these resistance bands will be similar to what you can get out of traditional weights or other machines. You don't have to use those complicated machines to get these resistance bands to work for you although you could add them to your workout if you wanted.

The muscles that you will work on when using these resistance bands can include all types of muscles on all parts of your body. You can use resistance bands to work on your calves, your arms, your thighs and much more. The best part is that it's not going to be too hard to make a workout run as the movements you can use are easy to figure out.

Be sure to plan your workouts based on the exercises you want to use. Make sure the workouts are even and that you're targeting all parts of your body in the process. Review the processes that you've read about in this guide and feel free to test them out to see if you can handle them. It can be a challenge for you to complete all of these tasks at first but over time you can strengthen and tone your body to where it will actually complete many of these movements.

The best part of working with resistance bands is that they are easy to manage and can come in many forms. You can add as much or as little resistance as you want.

Use this guide often to help you see what you can get out of your resistance bands. You will be amazed at how well a great resistance band workout can be to your advantage. This can especially be powerful for how you'll work with a variety of moves to make it effective.